A COMPLETE KETOGENIC DIET FOR BEGINNERS

Table of Contents

INTRODUCTION

In order to rapidly burn fat using the body's natural metabolism, consider a ketogenic diet plan. Nutrition has the strongest effect on the body's production of important hormones, which regulate metabolism and allow the body to burn fat for energy while retaining muscle mass, with little need for excessive exercise.

CHAPTER ONE:
KETO DIETING

What Is the Keto Diet?

The Keto diet involves going long spells on extremely low (no higher than 30g per day) to almost zero grams per day of carbs and increasing your fats to a really high level (to the point where they may make up as much as 65% of your daily macronutrients intake). The idea behind this is to get your body into a state of ketosis. In this state of ketosis, the body is supposed to be more inclined to use fat for energy- and research says it does just this. Depleting your carbohydrate/glycogen liver stores and then moving onto fat for fuel means you should end up being shredded.

Calculate your required maintenance level of daily calories...

(if you are looking to drop quickly, then use 13- I would not advise this, if you want a more level drop in body fat use 15, and if you are going to actually attempt to maintain or possibly put on some lean muscle mass, then use 17)

Body weight in pounds x 15= a

Protein for the day 1g per body weight in pounds= b

Bx4=c (c= number of calories allotted to your daily protein allowance)

a-c= d (d= amount of calories to be allotted to fat intake)

D/9= grams per day of fat to be consumed.

The end calculation should leave you with a very high number for your fat intake.

Now, for those of you wondering about energy levels... Especially for training because there are no carbs, with there being such a high amount of fat in the diet you will feel quite full and the fat is a very good fuel source for your body (one adaptation that I have made is to actually have a nice fish fillet about an hour before I train and I find it gives me enough energy to get through my workout).

I am aware of the arguments made to not have fats 2-3 hrs otherwise of training. While I won't have fats 2-3 hrs after training as I want quick absorption and blood flow, then I see no issue with slowing everything down before training so my body has access to a slow-digesting energy source.

Continuing with general guidelines...

There are some that say to have a 30g carb intake immediately after training- just enough to fill liver glycogen levels. And then there are those that say that having even as much as that may push you out of ketosis- the state you are trying to maintain.

During my carb up period- for the sake of those who would like to know if you can get in shape and still eat the things you want (in moderation)- for the first six weeks, I will be relaxed about what I eat in this period but then the following six weeks I only eat clean carbs.

I also like to make sure that the first workout of the week- as in a Monday morning workout- is a nice, long full hour of work so I start cutting into the liver glycogen already.

Plan menus and snacks at least a week ahead of time, so you aren't caught with only high-carb meal choices. Research keto recipes online; there are quite a few good ones to choose from. Immerse yourself in the keto lifestyle, find your favorite recipes, and stick with them.

There are a few items that are staples of a keto diet. Be sure to have these on hand:

- Eggs - Used in omelets, quiches (yes, heavy cream is legal on keto!), hard-boiled as a snack, low carb pizza crust, and more; if you like eggs, you have a great chance of success on this diet

- Bacon - Do I need a reason? Breakfast, salad garnish, burger topper, BLT's (no bread of course; try a BLT in a bowl, tossed in mayo)

- Cream cheese - Dozens of recipes, pizza crusts, main dishes, desserts

- Shredded cheese - Sprinkle over taco meat in a bowl, made into tortilla chips in the microwave, salad toppers, low-carb pizza and enchiladas

- Lots of romaine and spinach - Fill up on the green veggies; have plenty on hand for a quick salad when hunger pangs hit

- EZ-Sweetz liquid sweetener - Use a couple of drops in place of sugar; this artificial sweetener is the most natural and easiest to use that I've found

- Cauliflower - Fresh or frozen bags; you can eat this low-carb veggie by itself, tossed in olive oil and baked, mashed in fake potatoes, chopped/shredded and used in place of rice under main dishes, in low-carb and keto pizza crusts, and much more

- Frozen chicken tenders - Have a large bag on hand; thaw quickly and grill, saute, mix with veggies and top with garlic sauce in a low-carb flatbread, use in chicken piccata, chicken alfredo, tacos, enchiladas, Indian Butter chicken, and more

- Ground beef - Make a big burger and top with all sorts of things from cheese, to sauteed mushrooms, to grilled onions... or crumble and cook with taco seasoning and use in provolone cheese taco shells; throw in a dish with lettuce, avocado, cheese, sour cream for a tortilla-less taco salad

- Almonds (plain or flavored) - These are a tasty and healthy snack; however, be sure to count them as you eat, because the carbs DO add up. Flavors include habanero, coconut, salt and vinegar, and more.

The keto plan is a versatile and interesting way to lose weight, with lots of delicious food choices. Keep these 10 items stocked in your fridge, freezer, and larder, and you'll be ready to throw together some delicious keto meals and snacks at a moment's notice

SO WHAT FOODS ARE ENCOURAGED?

Some of the best-tasting, most fulfilling foods are part of this plan, including lean meats like beef and chicken; healthy sources of protein and high-quality fats like eggs, butter, olive oil, coconut oil, and avocado. Also, delicious, leafy, green vegetables like kale, chard, and spinach, as well as cruciferous vegetables like broccoli, cabbage, and cauliflower.

These foods can be combined with seeds, nuts, sprouts, and a wide range of other amazing foods that lead to incredible health benefits that give your body the protein, healthy fats, and nutrients it needs while providing metabolism-boosting meals for easy cooking at home or on the go.

WHAT FOODS SHOULD BE LIMITED?

On a ketogenic diet plan, the main foods to avoid are those high in carbohydrates, sugars, and the wrong types of fats. These foods can be toxic to the body and create excess glucose levels that the body turns into stored fat. These foods increase the levels of insulin and blood sugar in the body, and will prevent fat loss even if you are putting a lot of energy into exercise. To avoid these foods, limit your intake of grains, processed foods, vegetable oils (canola, corn, soybean, etc.), milk, margarine, and other high-carbohydrate, high-sugar foods.

WHAT ARE THE BENEFITS OF A KETOGENIC DIET PLAN?

- Burn Stored Fat - By cutting out the high levels of carbohydrates in your diet that produce glucose (sugar), a ketogenic diet plan tells your body to burn stored fat by converting this fat into fatty acids and ketone bodies in the liver. These ketone bodies replace the role of glucose that was being filled by carbohydrates in the diet. This leads to a rapid reduction in the amount of fat stored in the body.

- Retain Muscle Mass - By including the right fats in your diet, a ketogenic diet plan provides your body with the energy it needs to convert existing fat stores into useful sugars and ketones (through gluconeogenesis), which are an essential source of energy for the brain, muscles, and heart. This has the added benefit of preserving muscle mass, because the healthy fat in the diet gives the body the energy it needs without having to tap into muscle protein to create more sugar. This creates the best of both worlds – you burn fat while maintaining muscle mass!

- Eliminate Excess Fat - Even better, if your body creates too many ketone bodies by converting existing fat, it will simply eliminate those ketones as a waste product, which means you will basically pee out any unwanted body fat!

- Reduce Appetite - Lastly, by regulating the powerful metabolic hormones in your body, a ketogenic diet plan will actually reduce your appetite. By lowering your body's insulin resistance and increasing ketones, you will actually feel less hungry on this diet, which is an amazing advantage over other low-calorie, carbohydrate-rich weight loss diets that come with the expectation of lingering hunger.

Start burning fat today without more exercise! Take control of your metabolism naturally by adopting a ketogenic diet plan. Your body was designed for this style of nutrition. Your metabolic state can be optimized by consuming the (delicious) foods that our genetic forefathers thrived on, and this does not include carbohydrate-rich, processed foods loaded with sugars and bad fats. It involves a luxurious and fulfilling diet based on bountiful foods from paleolithic times, including lean meats, vegetables, nuts and seeds, and healthy fats that your body will thank you for

CHAPTER TWO:
KETOGENIC DIETS

Some would argue that only the first "phase" of the Atkins Diet is "ketogenic", but it's very clear that this element is central to the whole diet. There are many other diets of this type with different names and claims but, if they talk about severely restricting the intake of carbohydrates, then they're probably forms of a ketogenic diet. The process of "ketosis" is quite complicated and would take some time to describe but, in essence, it works because cutting down on carbs restricts the amount of blood glucose available to trigger the "insulin response". Without a triggering of the glucose-insulin response, some hormonal changes take place which cause the body to start burning its stores of fat as energy. This also has the interesting effect of causing your brain to be fuelled by what are known as "ketone bodies" (hence "ketogenic") rather than the usual glucose. The whole process is really quite fascinating and I recommend that you read up on it.

Controversy

All forms of ketogenic diet are controversial. Most of the debate surrounds the issue of cholesterol and whether ketogenic diets increase or decrease the levels of HDL "good" cholesterol and/or increase or decrease LDL "bad" cholesterol. The number of scientific studies is increasing year on year and it is certainly possible to point to strong cases on both sides of the argument. My conclusion (and this is only my opinion) is that one could equally make the case that a carbohydrate-laden diet has negative effects on cholesterol and I think that, on balance, a ketogenic-type diet is more healthy than a carbohydrate-heavy one. Interestingly, there isn't so much controversy about whether ketogenic diets work or not (it's widely accepted that they do); it's mostly about how they work and whether if that is good/bad/indifferent from a health perspective.

1. Low carb (ketogenic) diets deplete the healthy glycogen (the storage form of glucose) stores in your muscles and liver. When you deplete glycogen stores, you also dehydrate, often causing the scale to drop significantly in the first week or two of the

diet. This is usually interpreted as fat loss when it's actually mostly from dehydration and muscle loss. By the way, this is one of the reasons that low carb diets are so popular at the moment - there is a quick initial, but deceptive drop in scale weight.

Glycogenesis (formation of glycogen) occurs in the liver and muscles when adequate quantities of carbohydrates are consumed - very little of this happens on a low carb diet.

Glycogenolysis (breakdown of glycogen) occurs when glycogen is broken down to form glucose for use as fuel.

2. Depletion of muscle glycogen causes you to fatigue easily, and makes exercise and movement uncomfortable. Research indicates that muscle fatigue increases in almost direct proportion to the rate of depletion of muscle glycogen. Bottom line is that you don't feel energetic and you exercise and move less (often without realizing it) which is not good for caloric expenditure and basal metabolic rate (metabolism).

3. Depletion of muscle glycogen leads to muscle atrophy (loss of muscle). This happens because muscle glycogen (broken down to glucose) is the fuel of choice for muscles during movement. There is always a fuel mix, but without muscle glycogen, the muscle fibers that contract, even at rest to maintain muscle tone, contract less when glycogen is not immediately available in the muscle. Depletion of muscle glycogen also causes you to exercise and move less than normal, which leads to muscle loss and the inability to maintain adequate muscle tone.

Also, in the absence of adequate carbohydrates for fuel, the body initially uses protein (muscle) and fat. the initial phase of muscle depletion is rapid, caused by the use of easily-accessed muscle protein for direct metabolism or for conversion to glucose (gluconeogenesis) for fuel. Eating excess protein does not prevent this because there is a caloric deficit.

When insulin levels are chronically too low, as they may be in very low carb diets, catabolism (breakdown) of muscle protein increases, and protein synthesis stops.

4. Loss of muscle causes a decrease in your basal metabolic rate (metabolism). Metabolism happens in the muscle. Less muscle and muscle tone means a slower metabolism, which means fewer calories burned 24 hours-a-day.

5. Your muscles and skin lack tone and are saggy. Saggy muscles don't look good, cause saggy skin, and cause you to lose a healthy, vibrant look (even if you've also lost fat).

6. Some proponents of low-carb diets recommend avoiding carbohydrates such as bread, pasta, potatoes, carrots, etc. because they are high on the glycemic index - causing a sharp rise in insulin. Certain carbohydrates have always been, and will always be the bad guys: candy, cookies, baked goods with added sugar, sugared drinks, processed/refined white breads, pastas, and rice, and any foods with added sugar.These are not good for health or weight loss; carbohydrates such as fruits, vegetables, legumes, whole grain

breads and pastas, and brown rice are good for health and weight loss. Just like carbohydrates should be eaten in moderation. Large volumes of any proteins, fats, or carbohydrates are not conducive to weight loss and health.

The effect of high-glycemic foods is often exaggerated. It does matter, but to a smaller degree than is often portrayed. Also,the total glycemic effect of foods is influenced by the quantity of that food that you eat in a sitting. Smaller meals have a lower overall glycemic effect. Also, we usually eat several types of food at the same time, thereby reducing the average glycemic index of the meal, if higher glycemic foods are eaten.

Also, glycemic index values can be misleading because they are based on a standard 50 grams of carbohydrate consumed.

It wouldn't take many candy bars to get that, but it would take four cups of carrots. Do you usually eat four cups of carrots in a meal?

Regular exercisers and active people also are less affected by higher glycemic foods because many of the carbohydrates comsumed are immediately used to replenish glycogen stores in the liver and muscle.

By the way, if you're interested in lowering insulin levels, there is a great way to do that - exercise and activity.

7. Much of the weight loss on a low-carb, high-protein diet, especially in the first few weeks, is actually because of dehydration and muscle loss.

8. The percentage of people that re-gain the weight they've lost with most methods of weight loss is high, but it's even higher with low-carb, high-protein diets. This is primarily due to four factors:

    - You have lost muscle. With that comes a slower metabolism, which means fewer calories are burned 24 hours-a-day. A loss of muscle during the process of losing weight is almost a guarantee for re-gaining the lost weight, and more.

- You re-gain the healthy fluids lost because of glycogen depletion.

- It's difficult to maintain that type of diet long-term.

- You have not made a change to a long-term healthy lifestyle.

9. Eating too much fat is just not healthy. I know you've heard of people whose blood levels of cholesterol and triglycerides have decreased while on a low-carb, high-protein diet. This often happens with weight loss, but it doesn't continue when you're on a diet high in fat.

There are literally reams of research over decades that clearly indicate that an increase in consumption of animal products and/or saturated fat leads to increased incidence of heart disease, strokes, gall stones, kidney stones, arthritic symptoms, certain cancers, etc. For example, in comparing countries with varying levels of meat consumption, there is a direct relationship between the volume of meat consumption in a country and the incidence of digestive cancers (stomach, intestines, rectal, etc.).

CHAPTER THREE:
TYPES OF KETOGENIC DIETS

A ketogenic diet is a high-fat low-carbohydrate diet with adequate protein thrown in the meal. It is further divided into three types and, depending on one's daily calorie needs, the percentage differs. Diets are often prepared on a ratio level such as 4:1 or 2:1 with the first number indicating the total fat amount in the diet compared to the protein and carbohydrates combined in each meal.

Standard - SKD

The first diet is the Standard or the SKD and is designed for individuals who are not active or lead a sedentary lifestyle. The meal plan limits the dieter to eat a net of 20-50 grams of carbohydrates. Fruits or vegetables that are starchy are restricted from the diet. In order for the diet to be effective, one must strictly follow the meal plan. Butter, vegetable oil, and heavy creams are used heavily to replace carbohydrates in the diet.

Targeted - TKD

The TKD is less strict than the SKD and allows one to consume carbohydrates, though only in a certain portion or amount which will not impact the ketosis that one is currently in. The TKD diet helps dieters that perform some level of exercise or workout.

Cyclical - CKD

The CKD is preferable for those who are into weight training or do intensive exercises and is not for beginners as it requires the person undergoing the diet to stick to a SKD meal plan for five days in a week's time and eating/loading up on carbohydrates on the next two days. It is important that dieters follow the strict regimen to ensure that their diet is successful.

Ketones happen as a result of the body burning fat for energy versus glucose. A ketogenic diet refers to one that is low in carbohydrates, which will allow the body to break down fat faster in order to metabolize ketones.

Foods or ingredients that allow the body to make ketones are medium-chain triglycerides like:

- MCT oil

- Grass-fed butter

- Coconut oil

The important factor about ketones is that they help rid you of migraines.

HERE ARE THE TOP SEVEN WAYS KETONES SQUASH MIGRAINES:

1: Decreased Migraine Frequency

In recent studies, scientists have found that the ketogenic diet significantly reduced the frequency of migraines in 90% of patients. This completely dwarfs the effects of migraine drugs.

2: Glutamate Inhibition

Glutamate is found in both epilepsy and migraine patients. Medications that work in epilepsy (anti-seizure drugs) also block glutamate production. These drugs have been used to treat migraines as well. Since about 500 BC, ketones have worked to help prevent seizures, but the ketogenic diet has only been popular for the last century.

3: Processed Food

I have said many times that processed foods are bad for you, especially if you suffer with migraines. "Food-like products" are filled with preservatives, chemicals, and other triggers that could be affecting your migraine symptoms. Any diet that removes those processed foods, including the ketogenic diet, would be a good step to controlling migraine symptoms.

4: Saturated Fats

Several studies have debunked the great saturated fat myth. There are plenty of saturated fats (and other healthy fats) in a ketogenic diet, which has been found to reduce bad cholesterol and help the body produce serotonin and vitamin D, both of which help prevent migraines.

5: Hunger vs. Weight Management

Hunger is a major migraine trigger, so is weight gain/obesity. Some studies have found that weight gain and/or obesity increases the risk of migraines by 81%. Ketones help reduce hunger, while controlling insulin problems, promoting weight loss, and regulating glucose levels in the blood. Weight loss and sugar control are well-known benefits from adding MCT or coconut oil to your diet. Now, as you can see, they will help control migraines by helping you feel nutritionally satisfied, more energetic, improve cognitive functioning, and lose fat.

6: Oxidative Stress

A recent study found that oxidative stress is tied to migraine triggers. In response to these findings, a new migraine medication has come out which blocks the peptide released during oxidative stress. This drug also prevents glutamate release, another migraine trigger. You don't need to depend on medication, however. A ketogenic diet will do both for you, which indicates that ketones can not only treat migraine symptoms, but also determine the root cause.

7: MCT Oil

Research has found that Alzheimer's patients respond favorably to MCT (medium-chain triglyceride) oil, especially with regards to memory recall. Like Alzheimer's, migraine patients have white-matter brain lesions on their scans. Research in both diseases has found that ketones may help increase metabolism in the brain, even when oxidative stress and glucose intolerance is present.

Our minds and bodies need glucose and/or ketones to function and survive. We store about 24 hours' worth of sugar in our bodies, but we'd all die of hypoglycemia if not for the ketones. Metabolizing ketones from fat leaves our body in a healthy state of ketosis.

Migraines indicate that the brain is not metabolizing glucose into energy properly, so the logical response would be to add ketones. In addition to migraine pain symptoms, the ketogenic diet can help reduce:

- Brain fog

- Oxidative stress

- Brain lesions

A ketogenic diet can also help:

- Block glutamate (a major trigger)

- Eliminate processed foods (a major trigger)

- Add more saturated and healthy fats to your diet

- Control your weight

- Reduce oxidative stress

- Improve cognitive functioning

Chronic migraine headaches can control your life. The pain can be unbearable, relentless, and incredibly overwhelming, leaving you depressed, scared, and many times, alone.

CHAPTER FOUR:
KETOSIS - THE CYCLICAL KETOGENIC DIET BURN

We want to give a clearer picture of what your body will be going through while on the cyclical ketogenic diet. This chapter will focus on ketosis and what benefits it provides you.

Ketosis is a state in which your body goes on a fat-burning autopilot. How's that! The fat that is stored in your body begins to get used as energy, which will allow for weight reduction of fat, not water or muscle.

Many diets promoted are calorie-restriction diets. They help you lose weight, but, most of the weight is in the form of water and muscle. Little fat stores are broken down. This is the problem with a calorie-restrictive eating program. Your metabolism gets slower because your body begins to think it is starving and must slow down the process of losing calories. A slow metabolism equals slower weight loss and faster weight gain!

The cyclical ketogenic diet restricts carbohydrates. By restricting carbohydrates, but, maintaining caloric consumption, your body will have only one option of fuel consumption. That is fat; which is what ketosis is. You are essentially turning on your fat-burning machine. Ketones are sent out of your body and fat loss becomes profound. How does this happen? The largest internal organ in your body is the key player. Your liver. The liver has the job of converting fat into ketones. These ketones are then excreted out of the body, promoting weight/fat loss. This is a natural process.

Ketones are created in the liver and are an efficient source of energy for the body. Fatty acids that are broken down from body fat are created in the liver as these ketones. Ketones can only be made present when there is a lack of sugar and glucose in the body. Carbohydrates contain both of these substances. It will always be difficult to lose weight on a high-carbohydrate based diet. On the ketogenic diet, the amount of sugar and glucose is reduced to the point where they are no longer the primary source of fuel to be burned in the bloodstream.

We should take a moment to talk about a couple of myths surrounding the ketogenic diet and whether it is healthy in the long term. Our bodies can perform in the state of ketosis and be healthy. This state of ketosis is a natural occurrence when the body is not using sugar and glucose. The human body has no problem operating in this state naturally. In other words, it is safe to burn the fat.

HOW DO YOU KNOW IF YOU ARE IN A FAT-BURNING STATE?

A simple walk to the drug store can answer that quickly. You can use ketone testing strips to check your level of ketosis. Simply capture a urine sample on the strips and check for a color change. The magic color to look for is a pink to purple result. Check the color scale to see your ketone levels and where you are in the fat-burning zone.

The use of these strips will be your source of the level of ketones being released. This is the gauge by which you will know if you are properly keeping your carbohydrate intake to the necessary level to facilitate ketosis. Don't worry if you are not at the dark purple level. Different people have different levels. Just watch the scale and if you are losing weight, you are pretty much ok!

Here is a word of warning about dehydration. If you are seeing dark purple consistently, please make sure you are drinking enough water. Sometimes the dark purple indicates dehydration. Make sure you keep yourself hydrated properly when on the ketogenic plan.

The fat-burning mechanism associated with ketosis is at the heart of the cyclical ketogenic diet. Restricting carbohydrates and allowing your body the ability to burn those fat reserves will help you achieve your weight loss goals and obtain the body contour you have set goals to have. Get your ketone strips and watch your fat-burning begin.

Eat your veggies (they're the good carbs and won't interfere with your low carb benefits)!

Choose lean meats and eggs (eggs are a great source of protein, as is grass-fed organic meat)

Choose better fats (make sure you eat a regular supply of omega 3 fats amongst your other daily intakes. Saturated fat in moderation is not the danger. Sugar is)

Stay away from sugars and grains (low carbohydrate is less about maligning one particular food group and more about staying away from those sources which your body can't handle in large amounts)!

Athletes and healthy individuals may be able to use limited sugar and/or grains to improve performance but the same basic rules apply elsewhere)

Drink lots of water (we often argue over what groups of food are essential or not, but one we can all agree on is water. You need it and lots of it. Forget food, without water you die fast!)

Be wary of special low-carb foods (there are a great number of healthy choices here, athletes especially will enjoy easy-to-mix carb-free protein drinks, etc., but as low-carb diets have hit certain food industries hard, expect lots of products that may be lower carb choices but are not healthy. Always remember the low-fat craze where manufacturers swapped saturated fat for lots of sugar...)

Mix your food choices (restricting grains and sugars is a great start but don't fall into the trap of just surviving on the same meat diet day in and day out. Mix your proteins and fats and vegetables to offer a wide variety of healthy options)

Enjoy the diet (just because you stopped eating chips and bread with your meals doesn't mean you have to get bored! There is a limitless supply of sauces, seasonings, meats, eggs, and vegetables that don't require high-carb sugar and corn syrup additives to make great-tasting meals. Get fitter and healthier and enjoy your food while you do. Enjoying bacon once in a while poses little threat. Compare this to downing a fizzy drink with eight spoons of addictive, toxic sugar, and you see the advantages already)

CHAPTER FIVE:
LOW-CARB AND KETO DIET FAST FOOD MENU CHOICES

For those who eat low-carb or keto diets, there is almost always something you can eat in every fast food place or restaurant. Plan ahead. Before entering a restaurant, check out their menu and nutrition information online at home or using your smartphone. It's always good to know the safe options before being tempted by menu items you shouldn't have on a low-carb diet.

In order to make it easier to find a quick, keto-friendly option, I've compiled a list of several restaurants and fast food places and those items that I've found to be the lowest carb (and most emotionally satisfying) choices. These are not all perfect options, but when you're stuck with no other choices due to time or location constraints, they'll do in a pinch.

It's a huge help that fast-food places are required to post nutritional content. It gets easier to follow the keto plan every day. The carb count I'm listing is approximate and is NET grams.

In general, there is usually some sort of salad option anywhere you are. At burger joints, just remove the bun, and many places offer lettuce wraps instead. Chicken shouldn't have breading.

As a side note, it helps to have a knife and fork handy in your car or purse. Big, juicy burgers in tiny pieces of lettuce end up on the table - or in your lap. Small, flimsy fast food plasticware also makes for difficult eating. Pull out your own sturdy utensils and enjoy!

Now for the food choices... here are some pretty obvious general rules to follow:

Skip the bun or wrap

Skip the pasta, potato, or rice

Salads - No croutons. Stick with low-sugar dressing options - Caesar, Blue Cheese, Ranch, Chipotle. Look at the name which may give you a clue, things like "honey" in the honey dijon or "sweet" in the dressing name - these are usually not a good choice. Check the ingredients for items that are higher in carb content.

Chicken - Choose grilled or sauteed. Stay away from any chicken that is breaded.

Ketogenic Diet - Ultimate Fat Loss Diet

In simple terms, it's when you trick your body into using your own BODY FAT as its main energy source instead of carbohydrates. The keto diet is a very popular method of losing fat quickly and efficiently.

The Science Behind It

To get your body into a ketogenic state, you must eat a high-fat diet and low protein with NO carbs or hardly any. The ratio should be around 80% fat and 20% protein. This will be the guideline for the first two days. Once in a ketogenic state, you will have to increase the protein intake and lower fat; the ratio will be around 65% fat, 30% protein, and 5% carbs. Protein is increased to spare muscle tissue. When your body intakes carbohydrates, it causes an insulin spike which means the pancreas releases insulin (helps store glycogen, amino acids, and excess calories as fat) so common sense tells us that if we eliminate carbs, then the insulin will not store excess calories as fat. Perfect.

Now that your body has no carbs as an energy source it must find a new one. Fat. This works out perfectly if you want to lose body fat. The body will break down the body fat and use it as energy instead of carbs. This state is called ketosis. This is the state you want your body to be in, it makes perfect sense if you want to lose body fat while maintaining muscle.

Now to the diet part and how to plan it. You will need to intake AT LEAST a gram of protein per pound of LEAN MASS. This will help in the recovery and repair of muscle tissue after workouts and such. Remember the ratio? 65% fat and 30% protein. Well, if you weight 150 pounds of lean mass, that means 150g of protein a day, X4 (amount of calories per gram of protein), which is 600 calories. The rest of your calories should come from fat. If your caloric maintenance is 3000, you must eat around 500 less, which would mean that if you need 2500 calories a day, and around 1900 calories must come from fats! You must eat fats to fuel your body, which in return will also burn off body fat! That is the rule of this diet, you must eat fats! The advantage to eating dietary fats and the keto diet is that you will not feel hungry. Fat digestion is slow, which works to your advantage and helps you feel 'full'.

You will be doing this Monday - Friday and will then '' carb-up '' on the weekend. After your last workout on Friday, this is when the carb-up starts. You must intake a liquid carbohydrate along with your whey shake post workout. This helps create an insulin spike and helps get the nutrients your body desperately needs for muscle repair and growth and refill glycogen stores. During this stage (carb-up), eat what you want - pizzas, pasta, crisps, ice cream. Anything. This will be beneficial for you because it will refuel your body for the upcoming week, as well as restoring your body's nutrient needs. Once Sunday starts, it's back to the no-carb, high-fat, moderate protein diet. Keeping your body in ketosis and burning fat as energy is the perfect solution.

Another advantage to ketosis is that once your get into the state of ketosis and burn off the fat, your body will be depleted of carbs. Once you load up with carbs, you will look as full as ever (with less body fat!), which is perfect for the occasions on weekends when you go to the beach or parties!

Now let's recap on the diet.

- Must enter the state of ketosis by eliminating carbs from the diet while intaking high-fat moderate/low-protein.

- Must intake fibre of some sort to keep your pipes as clear as ever, if you know what I mean.

- Once in ketosis, protein intake must be at least that of a gram of protein per pound of lean mass.

Keto and Low-Carb Recipe Ideas: 5 Delicious Pizzas for Low-Carb and Keto Dieters

You can still eat pizza on the keto diet plan, but it takes a bit of creativity. When dining out, order a thin-crust pizza, then take your fork and slide all the toppings off the crust. It helps to order a pizza with lots of toppings. Ordering one topping on a deep dish pizza leaves you with very little left to eat.

As with most food options on keto, the best pizza is the one you make yourself. Try the low-carb pizza crust recipe, then use some of these ideas for toppings:

Mexican pizza - Use either traditional (low-carb) pizza sauce or enchilada sauce and top with taco-seasoned ground beef or chicken. Add a bit of salsa, chopped onions, chopped jalapeno peppers, and some hot sauce (Taco Bell hot sauce is the lowest in carbs). For some added flavor, add chopped cilantro. And top with sliced avocado after baking.

Greek pizza - Sauce, feta cheese, red onions, olives, and how about some artichoke hearts?

Buffalo chicken pizza - Frank's red-hot buffalo wing sauce is low in carbs. If you like hot, hot, hot, use chopped grilled chicken, some onions, crumbled blue cheese, and the buffalo sauce to make a zesty pizza. Don't forget to drizzle a little blue cheese dressing over the top.

Indian pizza - There's a local restaurant nearby that specializes in Indian pizzas,. If you choose to make this delicious option, you could use a packaged Indian food seasoning for chicken on top of the low-carb crust and add some veggies. If you want to start from scratch, season some chicken with traditional

Indian spices, like masala, curry powder, cumin, and any other spicy Indian seasonings you can think of. Add veggies, if desired.

Alfredo pizza - Use a keto diet-friendly Alfredo sauce or just spoon some out of a jar. Top with chicken or shrimp, plus garlic, parsley, Roma tomatoes - and extra parmesan cheese if you'd like.

KETOGENIC DIETS FOR MANAGING TYPE 2 DIABETES

Meat lovers - Pepperoni, sausage, bacon, pork, whatever you'd like. All these are very low-carb options.

Veggie lovers - Mushrooms, onions, tomatoes, all types of peppers, artichoke hearts... you name it, it'll taste great.

Three (or four, or five) cheese pizza - Try feta cheese, blue cheese, goat cheese, cream cheese, or any other tangy cheese, in addition to -- or in place -- of the traditional shredded mozzarella (remember, many low-carb crusts are also made out of cheese. You may want to be careful with overdoing it!).

Ketogenic diets have been in use since 1924 in pediatrics as a treatment for epilepsy. A ketogenic (keto) diet is one that is high in fat and low in carbs. The design of the ketogenic diet is to shift the body's metabolic fuel from burning carbohydrates to fats. With the keto diet, the body metabolizes fat, instead of sugar, into energy. Ketones are a byproduct of that process.

Over the years, ketogenic diets have been used to treat diabetes. One justification was that it treats diabetes at its root cause by lowering carbohydrate intake leading to lower blood sugar, which in turn, reduces the need for insulin, which minimizes insulin resistance and associated metabolic syndrome. In this way, a ketogenic diet may improve blood glucose (sugar) levels, while at the same time reducing the need for insulin. This point of view presents keto diets as a much safer and more effective plan than injecting insulin to counteract the consumption of high-carbohydrate foods.

A keto diet is actually a very restrictive one. In the classic keto diet, for example, one gets about 80% of caloric requirements from fat and 20% from proteins and carbohydrates. This is a marked departure from the norm, where the body runs on energy from sugar derived from carbohydrate digestion, but by severely limiting carbohydrates, the body is forced to use fat instead.

A ketogenic diet requires a healthy food intake from beneficial fats, such as coconut oil, grass-pastured butter, organic pastured eggs, avocado, fish such as salmon, cottage cheese, avocado, almond butter, and raw nuts (raw pecans and macadamia). People on ketogenic diets avoid all bread, rice, potatoes, pasta, flour, starchy vegetables, and dairy. The diet is low in vitamins, minerals, and nutrients and requires supplementation.

A low-carbohydrate diet is frequently recommended for people with type 2 diabetes because carbohydrates turn into blood sugar, and in large quantities they cause blood sugar to spike. Thus, for a diabetic who already has high blood sugar, eating additional sugar-producing foods is like courting danger. By switching the focus from sugar to fat, some patients can experience reduced blood sugar.

Changing the body's primary energy source from carbohydrates to fat leaves behind the byproduct of fat metabolism, ketones in the blood. For some diabetic patients, this can be dangerous, as a buildup of ketones may create a risk for developing diabetic ketoacidosis (DKA). DKA is a medical emergency requiring the immediate attention of a physician. DKA signs include consistently high blood sugar, dry mouth, polyuria, nausea, breath that has a fruit-like odor, and breathing difficulties. Complications can lead to diabetic coma.

HOW TO FOLLOW A PLANT-BASED KETOGENIC DIET

So, how exactly do you slip into ketosis without loading up on butter and bacon? And how can you ensure that your nutrient needs are still being met while following a plant-based ketogenic diet?

The key is to swap out your starchy veggies for low-carb alternatives, while also filling your diet with plenty of plant-based fats and proteins. This can help you stay under your carbohydrate goal and provide your body with the important vitamins and minerals that it needs to stay healthy.

High-carb foods that should be limited in your diet include:

- High-sugar fruits (apples, oranges, bananas, grapes, etc.)

- Starchy vegetables (potatoes, sweet potatoes, winter squash, peas, corn, etc.)

- Sugar (including honey, maple syrup, agave syrup, etc.)

- Legumes (beans, lentils, peas, etc.)

- Grains (wheat products, rice, quinoa, cereal, etc.)

Instead, be sure to include plenty of nutrient-rich, low-carb, plant-based foods in your diet, such as:

- Fermented foods (tempeh, natto, etc.)

- Leafy greens (kale, chard, spinach, collard greens, etc.)

- Non-starchy vegetables (asparagus, carrots, cauliflower, onions, mushrooms, peppers, etc.)

- Nuts (almonds, walnuts, pistachios, pecans, etc.)

- Seeds (chia seeds, flax seeds, hemp seeds, pumpkin seeds, etc.)

- Low-sugar fruits (blackberries, raspberries, strawberries, etc.)

- Healthy fats (coconut oil, MCT oil, olive oil)

Including enough protein in your diet can be challenging on any plant-based diet, let alone a plant-based ketogenic diet. Fortunately, there are tons of healthy options that can provide the protein you need to keep you going.

A few examples of low-carb, plant-based proteins include:

- Tempeh

- Natto

- Nutritional Yeast

- Spirulina

- Nuts

- Seeds

- High-quality, low-sugar plant-based protein powders

Similarly, nixing all dairy products from your diet can make it tricky to get in enough fat, but there are plenty of plant-based sources of fat available that can help you easily meet your needs.

Some of the healthiest plant-based fats include:

- Avocado Oil

- Coconut Oil

- Olive Oil

- MCT Oil

- Avocado

- Nuts

- Seeds

Note that you can easily swap these nutritious foods into your favorite recipes to make them completely plant-based and keto-friendly. Nutritional yeast, for example, makes a great substitute for cheese, while tempeh can be crumbled and cooked like ground beef to make delicious veggie tacos or lettuce wraps.

Sample Meal Plan:

Wondering what exactly a plant-based ketogenic diet looks like? Here's a one-day sample meal plan that you can follow to help get you started!

Breakfast:

Gluten-free oatmeal (2 grams net carbs per serving)

Lunch:

Baked tempeh (3 grams net carbs per serving)

Cauliflower tabbouleh salad (6 grams net carbs per serving)

Olive oil vinaigrette (0 grams net carbs per serving)

Dinner:

Raw walnut tacos (4 grams net carbs per serving)

Super cilantro guacamole (5 grams net carbs per serving)

Snacks:

Keto smoothie with avocado, chia seeds and cacao (6.5 grams net carbs)

Almonds (2.5 grams net carbs per 1-oz serving)

Spicy roasted pumpkin seeds (10 grams carbs per 1-oz serving)

Daily Total: 39 grams net carbs

CHAPTER SIX:
WHAT A VEGAN CAN EAT ON THEIR KETO JOURNEY

But can a vegetarian or vegan be keto? Does the necessity of fat and the small margin for carbs eliminate anyone else for meat and dairy consumers? No. Vegetarians and vegans can still be LCHF while observing their food preferences. Here at Keys to Ketosis, we've provided a vegan ketogenic diet food list to help anyone who is conscious of what types of food they consume, but still wants to (or has to) pursue a low-carb, high-fat lifestyle.

Check out the list of compiled low-carb vegan diet foods below

Tofu

The point of tension for a vegan/vegetarian attempting to pursue a LCHF will be the choices for a base food or "main course" food that will provide much of their protein and fat sources.

On the vegan ketogenic diet food list, Tofu will be one of the big operators for finding interesting ways to create mindful foods that also assist you in your low-carb pursuit. Tofu is a versatile food, that comes in various forms and can be cooked in a variety of ways, including grilling, frying, baking, or just eating it raw. Having this on your vegan ketogenic diet food list will be imperative to maintaining excitement and variety.

Tofu Nutriton Facts (1/2 Cup):

Calories: 94

Fats: 6g

Carbs: 2.3g

Protein: 10g

Nuts

Nuts are a must on the ketogenic diet, but peanuts should be eaten judiciously, due to their classification of legume, which means they belong to the same family as beans, and share their high-carb profiles. However, you can use peanut butter for a topping, but once again, not in excess.

The good news for your vegan ketogenic diet food list is that there are plenty of nuts that are permissible – and beneficial – due to being low-carb high-fat.

The best of the best include the following (in descending order from best to worst):

- Almonds

- Macadamia Nuts

- Walnuts

- Pecans

- Cashews and Pistachios

Nut-based flours can also be used for baking instead of high-carb wheat flour.

MCT Oil

MCT oil will make staying LCHF on a vegan diet easier than it has ever been.

MCT oil for the keto diet plan

By using this supplement in shakes, as a dressing, or on other foods, you can ensure that your body is getting the correct doses of fatty acids that are essential to ketosis.

Other ideas:

Mixing in toppings (like mayo)

Use while baking food instead of regular baking oil

The great thing about using MCT oil (and other exogenous ketones) is that you can counterbalance some of the carbs you will inevitably take by adhering to the vegan ketogenic diet food list.

Olive and Coconut Oil

Other oils that are great for toppings or cooking are coconut and olive oil. Both of these oils provide a great source of healthy fats, and a broad range of uses for food.

Olive oil in the vegan ketogenic diet food list

And unlike MCT oil, these oils can be used for frying and sautéing food. Coconut oil is more stable than olive oil, so it is the better choice for using at high temperatures.

Vegan ketogenic diet food list uses coconut oil

The benefit that these two oils bring to your vegan ketogenic diet food list, is their ability to provide vibrancy with flavor. While MCT oil can provide a more potent shot of healthy fat, it can also bring with it a taste that can be hard to handle if not masked, whereas coconut and olive oil are both pleasurable to consume.

Greens

Since fruits are a no on the ketogenic diet (except for avocados), you will need to be strategic about eating enough greens to get the nutrients you'd obtain from the fruits you'd normally consume on a standard vegan diet.

Leafy greens on the vegan ketogenic diet food list

The vegetables that you should keep stocked on your ketogenic diet food list are leafy greens like kale, collard greens, spinach, swiss chard, and others of the same family.

These vegetables, mixed with avocados and keto-friendly oils (listed above) will help you stay vibrant from proper vitamin intake, while also helping you maintain a low-carb lifestyle.

Fatty Produce (Avocado)

The avocado is the hallmark of healthy fats from fruits (yes, avocados are a fruit). It is also capable of being used in every meal of the day, pairing well with salads. Did we mention that guacamole is incredible?

Avocado in the vegan ketogenic diet food list

Avocados are considered a superfood, because research suggests they help lower cholesterol, and even ward off cancer!

Nutrition Info (1 avocado):

Calories: 322

Fats: 29g

Carbs: 17g

Protein: 4g

SOME MYTHS ON LOW-CARB DIETS

MYTH: Low carb diets are bad for health

Although pretty much all dietitians agree that cutting out sugar and refined flour is a good idea, there is still no consensus about low-carb nutrition amongst professionals. There are many scientific studies that show low-carb dieting to be not only not dangerous, but actually good for your health in many ways beyond weight loss. Specifically, it has been found that following some low-carb diet plans can improve digestion and levels of cholesterol.

Quite often, dietitians who don't specialise in low-carb nutrition (and so don't necessarily know much about it) have a knee-jerk negative reaction when asked about low-carb diets. For example, they often cite possible lack of vitamins as a negative factor. This is simply not true. Most low-carb diets do allow plenty of vegetables, and in fact, some people find that low-carb dieting means they start eating more vegetables, since that's their only permitted source of carbs.

However, as is the case with nutrition in general - whether trying to lose weight or not - it is important to be sensible and follow a plan that's been developed and tested by experts. If you suddenly stop eating all carbs and try to live on steak, cheese, and bacon, then clearly that would not be good for you. Contrary to the negative stereotype, this is not at all what low-carb dieting is all about. Choose a low-carb diet to suit your lifestyle, and then get the book and read it, so that you know exactly how to devise and manage your diet plan.

MYTH: Ketosis is dangerous

Being in ketosis means that fat is processed for energy instead of carbohydrates. Millions of people have experienced this state without any adverse health effects. Ketogenic diets are prescribed by mainstream medical professionals for managing symptoms of some diseases such as epilepsy.

Ketosis is sometimes confused with ketoacidosis, which is indeed a dangerous state but it only affects people with type 1 diabetes.

MYTH: Low-carb is not a natural way to eat

In fact, what's really unnatural is the standard Western diet that is high in refined sugar and flour.

Typical high-carb foods that are so abundant today are a result of technological advancement, and have only been available for the last century or two. There is nothing natural about white sugar - it is a result of a complicated refining process.

Going even further back, humans as a species have been hunters and fishers since long before they learned how to cultivate grains and other plant-based foods. Whatever plants or roots were available in those primitive societies, would have contained a lot less carbs than their modern-day counterparts, as they have by now been cultivated and bred selectively for centuries.

Finally, bear in mind that our lifestyles in the modern day are very different to those of our ancestors, even going back as early as a century ago. Technological progress means that most of us lead sedentary lives and do very little physical work. In developed countries, food is abundant and no one ever starves (sadly, this is not the case in some other areas of the world). Technology develops much too fast for a human body to evolve accordingly. Perhaps one day humans will evolve out of their basic need to consume and store food whenever they can. But in our lifetime, we will have to stick with diet and exercise to mitigate the consequences of food abundance.

MYTH: Low-carb dieters never get to eat any fruit or vegetables, and so may lack in vitamins

The myth about no fruit or vegetables is probably the most persistent one out there, and again, it is just simply not true. Most low-carb diets allow plenty of vegetables, and fruit is only restricted during the early phases of some plans.

Whilst there is no debate about vegetables, the way we think about fruit is actually sometimes misguided. We have come to think of them automatically as healthy, but in reality, some fruit are extremely high in sugar. Eating several oranges or a pack of grapes in one go gives you the same amount of sugar as a chocolate bar would. Whilst of course fruit would be better than chocolate (as it also contains fibre and vitamins), sugar is still sugar, and you should eat less of it if you want to lose weight. Fruit juices remove fibre from the fruit, and in fact are hardly better than sugary fizzy drinks.

If you are worried about getting enough vitamins in the early, more restrictive stages of your diet, consider taking a multivitamin supplement.

MYTH: Not getting enough carbs will make me tired

It is true that you may experience a short period of tiredness while your body adjusts. However, this period usually only lasts for several days. Once your body switches to burning fat instead of carbohydrates for energy, you are likely to find yourself feeling more energetic than before. Moreover, you will feel so on a consistent and continuous basis - in contrast to roller-coaster up and down energy levels typical of a high-carb diet.

CHAPTER SEVEN: INFLAMMATION - EATING ANTI-INFLAMMATORY FOODS

Are there really diets out there that can reduce inflammation? Do they work? Scientists have found that there is a relationship, in part, between what we eat and inflammation. They've even identified some compounds in food that can reduce inflammation and others that promote it. There is still a lot to learn about just how diet and inflammation interact, and research, as of yet, is not at that point where a specific foods or groups of foods can be singled out as being beneficial for people with, for example, arthritis. We are beginning to get a clearer picture of how eating the right way can reduce inflammation.

So why are we so concerned about inflammation? Inflammation is the body's natural defense to infections and injuries. When something goes wrong, the body's immune system goes to work to inflame the area, which serves to get rid of the invader or to heal the wound. Inflammation can cause pain, swelling, redness, and warmth, but this goes away as soon as the problem is solved. This is good inflammation.

Then we have chronic inflammation, the type that's familiar to people with rheumatoid arthritis (RA), lupus, psoriatic arthritis, and other types of "inflammatory" arthritis. Chronic inflammation is the type that will not go away. All the types of arthritis that are mentioned above are a disorder of the immune system which creates inflammation and then doesn't know when to shut off. Inflammatory arthritis' chronic inflammation can have serious consequences, permanent disability and tissue damage can be done if it isn't treated properly. Inflammation has been linked to a full host of other medical conditions.

Inflammation has been found to contribute to atherosclerosis, which is when fat builds up on the lining of arteries, raising the risk of heart attacks. Also, high levels of inflammation proteins have been found in the blood of people with heart disease. Inflammation has also been linked to obesity, diabetes, asthma, depression, and even Alzheimer's disease and cancer. Scientists think that a constant level of inflammation in the body, even if the level is low, can have a number of negative effects. Research shows that a diet can reduce inflammation; in theory an inflammation-lowering diet should have an effect on a wide range of health conditions.

Researchers have looked for clues in the eating habits of our early ancestors to discover which foods might benefit us the most. They believe those habits are more in tune to our eating habits with how the body processes and uses what we eat and drink. Our ancestors' diet consisted of wild lean meats (venison or boar) and wild plants (green leafy vegetables, fruits, nuts, and berries). There were no cereal grains until the agriculture revolution (about 10,000 years ago). There was very little dairy, and there were no processed or refined foods. Our diets are usually are high in meat, saturated (or bad) fats, and processed foods, and there is very little exercise. Nearly everything we eat is available close by or as far away as our computer and the click of a mouse.

Our diet and lifestyles are way out of whack with how our bodies are made from the inside out. While our genetic make-up has changed very little from our early beginnings, our diet and lifestyles have changed a great deal, and the changes have gotten worse over the last 50 to 100 years. Our genes haven't had a chance to adapt. We aren't giving our bodies the right kind of fuel, it's as though we think of our bodies as engines in a jet plane, when instead they are like the engine in the very first planes. There are some foods that we are putting into our bodies, especially because we are eating way too much of them, that are affecting our health in a bad way.

There are two nutrients in our diets that have attracted attention, which are omega-3 fatty acids and omega-6 fatty acids that have been part of our diets for thousands of years. They are components in just about all of our many cells and are important for normal growth and development. Both of these acids play a role in inflammation. In several studies it was found that certain sources of omega-3s in particular, help to reduce the inflammation process and that omega-6s will raise it.

Now this is the problem, the average American eats on average about 15 times more omega-6s than omega-3s. While our very early ancestor's ate omega-6s and omega-3s in equal ratio, and it is believed that this is what helped to balance their ability to turn inflammation on and off. The imbalance of omega-3s and omega-6s in our diets is believed to contribute to the excess of inflammation in our bodies.

So why is it that we eat so many omega-6s now? Vegetable oils such as corn oil, safflower oil, sunflower oil, cottonseed oil, soybean oil, and the products made from them, such as margarine, are loaded with omega-6s. Even many of the processed snack foods that are so readily available today are full of these oils. Based on the best information of the time, the best suggestion was to use vegetable oils like those mentioned above instead of foods with saturated fats such as butter and lard. It looks like the consequences of that advice may have contributed to the increased consumption of omega-6s and therefore caused an imbalance of omega-3s and omega-6s.

You can find omega-6s in other common foods such as meats and egg yolks. The omega-6 found in meat is the fatty acids that come from grain-fed animals such as cows, lambs, pigs, and chickens. Most of the meat sold in America is grain-fed, unlike their grass-fed cousins who contain less of those fatty acids.

Wild game such as venison and boar are lower in omega-6s and fat and higher in omega-3s than the meat that comes from the supermarkets where we shop.

You can get omega-3s in both animal and plant foods. Our bodies can convert omega-3s from animal sources into anti-inflammatory compounds more easily than the omega-3s from plant sources. Plant foods contain hundreds of other healthful compounds, many of which are anti-inflammatory, so don't discount them all together.

There are many foods that are high in omega-3s and those include fatty fish, especially fish from cold waters. Of course everyone knows about salmon, but did you know that you can also find omega-3s in mackerel, anchovies, sardines, herring, striped bass, and bluefish? It's also widely known that wild fish are better sources of omega-3s than farm-raised ones. You can also buy eggs that have been enriched with omega-3 oils. There are several excellent sources of omega-3s in plants that are leafy greens (like kale, Swiss chard, and spinach) as well as flaxseed, wheat germ, walnuts, and their oils.

You can also get omega-3s in supplements (often as fish oil); this source has been shown to be beneficial in some instances. You should talk with your doctor before you take a fish oil supplement because it can interact with some medications and under certain circumstances can increase the risk of bleeding. I take a prescribed omega-3 supplement because my doctor had told me that the ones you get in the supermarket or health food store are not pure, they have other additives that do absolutely nothing to help. There are other fats that are contributors to clogged arteries, the "bad" or saturated fats found in meats and high-fat dairy foods, which are called pro-inflammatory.

There are also the trans fats that are relatively new to the cause of heart disease. These trans fats can be found in processed convenience and snack foods and can be spotted by reading the labels. They can be identified as partially hydrogenated oils, often soybean oil or cottonseed oil. But, they can also occur naturally in small amounts in animal foods. The thought is that they contribute to the pro-inflammatory activities in our bodies and the amounts we eat today are staggering.

Antioxidants are substances that prevent inflammation, causing "free radicals" to overtake our bodies. Plant foods such as fruits, vegetables (including beans), nuts, and seeds carry high amounts of antioxidants. Extra-virgin olive oil and walnut oil are very good sources of antioxidants, as well. These foods have long been considered the basics for good health, and can be found in fruits and vegetables with colorful and vibrant pigments. The more colorful the plant, the better they are for you, from green vegetables, especially leafy ones, to low-starch vegetables, such as broccoli and cauliflower, to berries, tomatoes, and brightly-colored orange and yellow fruits and vegetables.

We don't have to revert back completely to the caveman to eat the anti-inflammatory way to benefit from the anti-inflammatory diet. Just eating a healthful diet that is recommended today is right on track. Our chief strategy should be to balance the amount of modern-day foods with those of long ago, which were rich in the inflammation reducing foods. Really, all we have to do is replace foods rich in omega-6 with foods rich in omega-3, cutting down on how much meat and poultry we eat while eating oily fish a couple of times a week and adding more varieties of colorful fruits and vegetables, and while whole grains were not a part of our early ancestor's diet, they should be included in ours. Be sure that it is whole grains and not refined grains because they contain many beneficial nutrients and inflammation-tempering compounds. Researchers have found that eating a lot of foods high in sugar and white flour may promote inflammation, although there is more studying that needs to be done on the subject.

The amounts of knowledge we have on how the body works and how our ancestors ate is helping to confirm the old adage: "You are what you eat." But, there is still more we need to learn before we can prescribe any one anti-inflammatory diet. Our genetic makeup and the severity of our health condition will determine the benefits we get from an anti-inflammatory diet and unfortunately there is doubt that there will be one regimen that fits us all.

Also, what we eat or don't eat is just a small part of the whole story. We are not as physically active as our ancestors and exercise has its own anti-inflammatory effects. Our ancestors were also much leaner than we are and body fat is active tissue that can make inflammatory producing compounds.

Anti-inflammatory eating is a way of selecting foods that are more in tune with what the body actually needs. We can achieve a more balanced diet by going back to our roots. If you look at the diet of the people of the Bible, you will find that they, like our caveman ancestors, were more active and their diets consisted of much the same things as our caveman ancestors. They also had no choice but to walk everywhere they wanted to go, there was no such thing as cars or trucks. While we have it easier today, our health has suffered greatly from it.

CHAPTER EIGHT:
KETOGENIC DIET FREQUENTLY ASKED QUESTIONS

Here are some answers to some of the most commonly asked questions...

Why do I keep reverting back to my old "out of shape" self?

You work out for a few months and get in shape and fall back to the old habits because you were not conditioned mentally, only physically. Physical fitness is only a part of journey, and fitness is over 75% percent mental. Gyms, nutritionists, and personal trainers give most people a temporary Band-Aid but never address the actual issue.

How do you know when your body is in ketosis?

Any of these signs may indicate you are in ketosis:

Decreased appetite and increased energy levels.

Increased thirst and urination.

"Keto breath", which may be more apparent to others than to yourself

Dry mouth or a metallic taste in your mouth.

Beyond these signs and symptoms, you can measure your level of ketosis, using one of three methods:

- Urine strips

- Breath analyzers

- Blood meters

What foods can you eat on a keto diet?

Eat real low-carb foods like meat, fish, eggs, vegetables, and natural fats (like olive oil or butter). A simple rule for beginners is to eat foods with fewer than 5% carbs

Is a keto diet safe for the kidneys?

Yes. People often wonder about this, because of the belief that a diet high in protein could be harmful for the kidneys. However, this fear is simply based on two misunderstandings:

A keto diet is high in fat, not protein.

People with normal kidney function handle excessive protein just fine.

Is ketosis safe for diabetics?

A keto diet leading to ketosis is generally a very powerful treatment to reverse type 2 diabetes.

People with type 1 diabetes can use a keto or low-carb diet to significantly improve their blood-sugar control. They will however normally always require insulin injections, but usually far lower doses on keto. They need to take care to not take too low doses and end up with ketoacidosis, or too high and end up with keto.

Both people with type 1 and type 2 may rapidly require a reduction in medication on a keto diet to avoid hypoglycemia.

How many carbs can you eat and still be in ketosis?

This varies, but generally it's a good idea to stay below 20 net carbs per day.

Some people who are not insulin-resistant – e.g. lean, young people who exercise regularly – can sometimes tolerate more carbs, perhaps 50 grams or more per day.

Is a ketogenic diet safe for high cholesterol?

Generally, the cholesterol profile tends to improve on a keto diet, lowering triglycerides and raising the good HDL cholesterol.

However, a small minority of people may end up with quite high total cholesterol. Whether this is dangerous or safe is debated – there are no quality studies to determine the answer. But should you be one of the few where cholesterol may get up very high, e.g. over 400, you may want to take steps to reduce it just to be safe.

Can I have fruit on a keto diet?

Although fruits are often considered healthy, they are actually very high in carbs and sugar, unlike non-starchy vegetables. Therefore, when it comes to keto diets, most fruits should be avoided.

However, certain berries are an exception that can be enjoyed in small amounts. The best choices are blackberries, raspberries, and strawberries, which provide 5-6 grams of carbs per 100 grams (3½ ounces).

Most other fruits – including blueberries – contain double or triple this amount of carbs, as reflected in this guide to the best and worst fruits in terms of carb content.

Keep in mind that berries don't provide any nutrients that can't be found in vegetables and other foods with fewer carbs, so they are entirely optional on a keto diet. In fact, if you are very insulin-resistant, you might be better off not having them.

How long can someone be on a keto diet?

As long as you want to, and enjoy it.

Can I eat a keto diet as a vegetarian or vegan?

A keto diet can work for many non-meat-eaters, depending on what other types of food their diets include.

A lacto-ovo vegetarian eats dairy and eggs, whereas a lacto-vegetarian eats dairy but doesn't eat eggs. There is also a subset of vegetarians known as pescatarians who include fish in their diet but avoid poultry and other meat.

Although following keto as a vegetarian is definitely doable, it can be a little challenging, especially when first starting out.

A keto vegetarian meal plan provides several well-balanced, healthy meat-free meals.

On the other hand, a ketogenic vegan diet isn't a well-balanced or sustainable option. Because vegans exclude all animal products, they must rely on a combination of grains, legumes, and seeds to get all the essential amino acids their bodies need. For this reason, a keto diet and vegan diet don't work well together. Therefore, you'll need to make a choice between the two or consider following a keto vegetarian diet.

What should my ketone level be in ketosis?

Generally above 0.5 mmol/l.

What can I do for keto breath?

How to handle keto breath.

Can I have dairy on keto?

Dairy is nutritious and can be part of a keto diet in many cases. However, whether you personally should eat dairy may depend on your health goals, along with your personal response to it.

For instance, although a higher dairy intake has been linked to fat loss and reduced diabetes risk in several studies, it has also been found to raise insulin levels. Indeed, some people find that cutting back on dairy helps with weight loss.

It's also important to avoid high-carb options typically considered "healthy," such as nonfat milk and nonfat yogurt. Instead, focus on these high-fat choices, preferably from naturally raised animals:

- Butter

- Cream

- Sour cream

- Cream cheese

- Cheese

- Plain whole-milk yogurt, Greek yogurt, or kefir

Can you build muscle on keto?

Yes.

What's the difference between low-carb and keto diets?

Keto is a very strict low-carb diet, that also puts even more emphasis on moderating the protein intake, and relying primarily on fat to supply energy needs.

A regular strict low-carb diet will likely put most people in ketosis anyway. But a keto diet tweaks things even further to make sure it's working and, if desired, to get even deeper into ketosis.

Keto could be called an extra strict low-carb diet.

Why am I not in ketosis?

The two most common reasons for not getting into ketosis are:

Too many carbs

Too much protein

Should you aim for high ketone levels to speed up weight loss?

Yes and no. Eating fewer carbs, less protein, and doing intermittent fasting certainly promotes weight loss, while lowering insulin and raising ketones.

However, adding extra fat to raise ketone levels does not promote weight loss. Neither does supplementing with MCT oil to raise ketone levels, or drinking "exogenous" ketone supplements. These methods actually slow down weight loss, by providing alternative fuel to be used instead of burning body fat.

If you want to lose weight, only use these methods – MCT oil or exogenous ketones – when you are hungry, or for performance reasons (unrelated to weight loss).

At what time of the day should you test ketone levels?

For comparison purposes, it's good to measure about the same time every day. Measuring in the morning before eating makes it easier to compare the result from day to day.

However, morning numbers are usually among the lowest of the day, while evening numbers are higher. So if for some reason you want impressively high numbers, measure in the evenings instead. Be aware that your ketone levels don't distinguish between the burning of dietary fat and stored fat.

Is keto safe during pregnancy?

A keto diet appears to be safe during pregnancy, judging from the experiences of people who have done it and doctors used to treating patients using a keto diet during pregnancy. It may also be very helpful in cases of gestational diabetes.

However, there are no scientific studies on the subject, so there is a lack of definite knowledge. Possibly it's wise to exercise caution and aim for a more moderate low-carb diet during pregnancy, unless there are important health benefits of doing a keto diet in your specific case.

How To Know If You're In Ketosis

You can measure if you're in ketosis via urine or blood strips, although it is pretty simple to just use physical indicators to tell if you are "spilling ketones."

Here is a list of "symptoms" that usually let you know if you're in a state of ketosis:

Increased Urination. Ketones act as a natural diuretic, so you have to go to the bathroom more. Acetoacetate, a ketone body, is also excreted in urination and can lead to increased bathroom visits for beginners.

Dry Mouth. The increased urination leads to dry mouth and increased thirst. Make sure that you're drinking plenty of water and replenishing your electrolytes (salt, potassium, magnesium).

Bad Breath. Acetone is a ketone body that partially excretes in our breath. It can smell sharp like overripe fruit, similar to nail polish remover. It's usually temporary and goes away after a short while.

Reduced Hunger and Increased Energy. After you get past the initial stages of the ketogenic diet and your body had adjusted, you'll experience a much lower hunger level and a "clear" or energized mental state.

Note: Many people end up driving themselves crazy measuring and testing! It's much better to focus on the nutritional aspect, making sure that you're consuming proper foods and staying within your macro ranges.

The Ketogenic Diet: Bottom Line

The Ketogenic Diet: Not only does the ketogenic diet help you to lose weight and alter your metabolic state, but it will also help you to become healthier overall by lowering your cholesterol and blood pressure, regulating your insulin levels, giving you more energy, eliminating unhealthy food cravings, and improving your mental performance.

Admittedly, the keto diet can be intimidating at first, but it is a truly empowering way of life once you grasp the concept and start seeing the results!

When you limit your carbohydrate intake you will primarily get your 15g of carbs or more a day from nuts, dairy, and vegetables. You will be encouraged to AVOID potatoes, beans, fruit, legumes, bread, pasta, cereal, and any sugar (refined carbs and starches).

There are a few exceptions to these foods once you have maintained ketosis for a while, such as berries and star fruit, and avocado can be consumed later in the diet in moderation.

Here are a few examples of the "do eat" and "do not eat" foods list for the keto diet:

Do Not Eat

- Grains – wheat, corn, rice, cereal, etc.

- Sugar – honey, agave, maple syrup, etc.

- Fruit – apples, bananas, oranges, etc.

- Tubers – potato, yams, etc.

Do Eat

- Meats – fish, beef, lamb, poultry, eggs, etc.

- Leafy Greens – spinach, kale, etc.

- Above ground vegetables – broccoli, cauliflower, etc.

- High Fat Dairy – hard cheeses, high fat cream, butter, etc.

- Nuts and seeds – macadamias, walnuts, sunflower seeds, etc.

- Avocado and berries – raspberries, blackberries, and other low glycemic impact berries, etc.

- Sweeteners – stevia, erythritol, monk fruit, etc.

LOW-CARB CHEESE CRACKERS RECIPE INGREDIENTS

Ingredients:

- 2 cups cheese of your choice (use a Parmesan-Romano mix along with some Swiss and cheddar)

- 1 cup almond flour

- 2 oz cream cheese

- 1 egg

- 1/2 teaspoon sea salt

- 1 teaspoon rosemary (or a seasoning of your choice such as basil, chives, garlic, dill weed, spicy chili, thyme, oregano etc...)

Instructions:

Mix all the cheeses (including the cream cheese) along with the almond flour in a microwave safe bowl and cook it for exactly one minute(there are some people that prefer not to use a microwave and I certainly understand that. You can heat these ingredients up on the stove top too. You are going to heat them up just enough for the cheese to my melted enough for you to roll out the dough. I would continue stirring it while heating it up on the stove top).

Immediately stir the ingredients until the almond flour and cheeses have combined fully. You want the cheese to be partially melted.

Allow this to cool for a few minutes because if you put the egg in these ingredients too soon it will cook the egg.

Now add the egg, sea salt, and seasoning of your choice. I decided to cut up some fresh rosemary I had on hand. You want to add about a teaspoon of your favorite seasoning unless it's a spicy mix. I would add only about a 1/2 teaspoon for spicy seasonings.

Mix it together until all the ingredients are fully combined. If you cheese has gotten too hard or it's too hard to mix, you can microwave your cheese for another 20 seconds to get it soft again.

Now you will place the ball of dough on a large sheet of parchment paper. Then place another sheet of parchment paper of equal size on top of the ball of dough.

You can use your hands or a rolling pin to spread the dough out into a thin layer. It spread so easily that I used my hands to have more control and keep the dough inside the square piece of parchment paper. Make sure the parchment paper is the same size as your baking sheet.

Next, use a pizza cutter to cut the crackers into small squares as seen in the photos.

Bake these crackers on each side at 450 degrees for about 5 or 6 minutes on each side. If the crackers are thin, you will cook them about 5 minutes on each side but if the dough is thick, it may take 7 to 9 minutes to get the crispy cracker texture you are looking for. When you keep the dough on the parchment paper it's really easy to flip it over while it's hot after cooking it on the first side.- Feel free to leave the crackers in the oven longer (but watch them closely) if you love a very crispy texture. The crispier the better for me!

Allow the crackers to cool for about 5 minutes and they are ready to eat!

INGREDIENTS FOR KETO PRETZELS:

Ingredients:

- 3 cups Mozzarella cheese, shredded

- 4 tablespoons of cream cheese

- 1 ½ cups of almond flour

- 2 teaspoons of xanthum gum

- 2 Eggs, at room temperature

- 2 teaspoons of dried yeast, approximately 1 sachet

- 2 tablespoons of warm water

- 2 tablespoons of butter, melted

- 1 tablespoon of pretzel salt

How To Make Keto Soft Pretzels:

Preheat oven to 200C/390F.

In a microwave safe dish, place the mozzarella cheese and cream cheese and microwave in 30 sec increments, stirring in between, until fully melted and almost liquid.

Dissolve the yeast in the warm water and allow it to sit and activate for 2 minutes.

In your stand mixer (using the dough hook attachment), place the almond meal and xanthum gum and mix well.

Add the eggs, yeast mixture and 1 tablespoon of the melted butter and mix well.

Add the hot melted cheese to the stand mixer and allow it to knead the dough until all the ingredients are fully combined. Around 5-10 minutes.

Split the dough into 12 balls. The dough is easiest to work with while it is warm.

Roll each ball into a long skinny log and twist into a pretzel shape. Place on a lined cookie sheet and give a little space with side as the pretzels will rise.

Brush the pretzels with the remaining butter and sprinkle with pretzel salt.

Bake in the oven for 12-15 minutes.

When the pretzels are golden brown, remove them from the oven. Don't burn your fingers trying to eat them immediately.

If you're looking for a sweet version of these keto pretzels try our glazed pretzels. Our glazed pretzels taste like a low-carb doughnut.

PALEO BROWNIES RECIPE

TOTAL TIME - 40 minutes

Ingredients:

- ½ cup coconut oil

- 2 eggs

- ⅓ cup dark chocolate chips

- ½–¾ cup maple sugar

- ¾ teaspoon Himalayan pink salt

- 3 tablespoons arrowroot starch

- ¼-½ cup cocoa or cacao powder

- 2 teaspoons vanilla

Instructions:

Preheat oven to 350 F.

Melt the coconut oil and chocolate chips in a small pot over medium heat.

Using a hand mixer, mix all the other ingredients together until the batter is thick.

Pour contents into a 8.5" X 4.5" X 2.75" loaf pan.

Bake for 30 minutes.

Allow to cool for 15 minutes.

Do you know what else? This Paleo brownie recipe is no harder or more time-consuming than a traditional brownie recipe. Plus, you loose nothing in the flavor department. This recipe includes dark chocolate chips, Himalayan pink salt, vanilla extract, coconut oil... Before you start making your delicious Paleo brownies, you'll need to preheat your oven to 350 F.

Next, in a small pot, after melting the coconut oil, add chocolate chips over medium heat.

Now you can start combining all of your other ingredients into a large mixing bowl, starting with sea salt and maple sugar...

Add the arrowroot starch...

–Stir in the vanilla extract.

Using a hand mixer, mix all the other ingredients together until the batter is thick.

Bake for 30 minutes.

I know it's hard to wait, but allow these delicious brownies to cool for 15 minutes before digging your teeth into one

STUFFED MUSHROOMS RECIPE

TOTAL TIME - 25 minutes

Ingredients:

- 1 tablespoon melted coconut oil, divided

- 20 cremini mushroom caps

- 1 package uncured turkey bacon

- 1 head of cauliflower, chopped

- ¼ cup grated raw goat cheese

- ½ teaspoon minced garlic

- 1 tablespoon sea salt

- 1 tablespoon pepper

- 2 tablespoons unsalted grass-fed butter, diced into 20 pieces

- ½ cup chives

Instructions:

Heat the oven to 400 F.

Brush the mushroom caps with the coconut oil and place them top down on a baking sheet.

Use the remaining oil to grease another baking sheet.

Distribute the bacon evenly on the greased baking sheet.

Bake the mushrooms and bacon for 15 minutes.

While the mushrooms and bacon are baking, bring a medium pot of water to a boil.

Add the cauliflower and boil for 8 minutes, or until tender.

Drain the cauliflower well and remove any excess water by patting with paper towels.

Do not allow the cauliflower to cool.

To the bowl of a food processor, add the cauliflower, cheese, garlic, salt and pepper and puree until almost smooth.

Set aside.

Remove the mushrooms and bacon from the oven.

Chop up the bacon.

Flip the mushroom caps and fill them with the cauliflower mixture.

Place one piece of butter on top of the mixture.

Crumble and sprinkle the bacon on top of each mushroom.

Serve immediately.

KETO BANANA WALNUT BREAD RECEPIE:

Ingredients:

- 3 Medium Bananas

- 2 Cups Almond Flour

- 3 Large Eggs

- 1/2 Cup Walnuts

- 1/4 Cup Olive Oil

- 1 Tsp Baking Soda

- Coconut Oil

Instructions:

Preheat oven to 350

Grease loaf pan using coconut oil

Cut up bananas

Add all ingredients in a mixing bowl and mix on high until well combined

Pour mix into loaf pan and bake for 50-60 minutes

Keto Banana Walnut Bread Recipe: Nutrition

This is for one serving (makes 10 servings)

PORRIDGE

Textured vegetable protein (dry soy granules) are usually used in savory recipes, but it actually has a neutral flavor which means they can also be used in sweet recipes! If you cook them with soy or almond milk, sweetener and some cinnamon, they actually taste quite similar to oatmeal, making a nice high protein low carb breakfast porridge

This recipe makes a single serving, but you can easily double or triple it etc. to make more. If you let the porridge cool down it will keep for a few days in the fridge. You can heat up a portion when you are hungry or even just eat it cold.

Ingredients:

- 1/3 cup tvp granules

- 2/3 cup unsweetened plant milk (for instance soy or almond)

- 1/4 teaspoon cinnamon

- low carb sweetener to taste

- optional: vanilla extract, nutmeg, fruit etc.

Instructions:

Put all the ingredients into a small pot and bring it to a boil. Turn down the heat and let it cook for 10-15 minutes, until the tvp is soft. Stir often so the porridge won't burn to the bottom of the pot. Eat it warm or let it cool down and eat it cold. It will keep for a few days in the fridge

GRANOLA WITH ALPRO SOY

Time: preparation 5 minutes,

Cooking 10 minutes

Total 15 minutes

Ingredients:

- 1 cup sunflower seeds

- 1/2 cup pumpkin seeds

- 1/2 cup shredded dried coconut

- concentrated liquid sweetener to taste (optional)

- 1/4 cup whole flax seed

- 1/4 cup ground flax seed

Instructions:

Preheat a skillet to medium high on your stove. Pour in the sunflower and pumpkin seeds and toast them until they start to turn golden brown. Stir well while toasting, so they don't burn.

Take the pan off the heat and and the shredded coconut. Stir in the sweetener until the granola is sweet enough for your taste.

Sprinkle in the whole and ground flax (don't do this earlier, or the flax will absorb the liquid sweetener, making it difficult to distribute it evenly over the granola).

Let the granola cool completely and transfer it to an airtight container. It will keep for at least a month in your pantry, and much longer in the fridge or freezer.

THAI PEANUT-PINEAPPLE FRIED RICE

Prep Time 15min.

Total Time 35min.

Put sweet and savory deliciousness on the menu with Thai Peanut-Pineapple Fried Rice. Thai Peanut-Pineapple Fried Rice is ready to eat in 35 minutes.

Ingredients:

- 1/4 cup teriyaki sauce

- 8 oz. firm tofu, cubed

- 1 Tbsp. PLANTERS Peanut Oil

- 1 red pepper, cut into strips

- 1/2 cup green onion pieces (1 inch)

- 2-2/3 cups cooked long-grain brown rice, chilled

- 1 can (8 oz.) pineapple tidbits in juice, drained

- 1/2 cup PLANTERS COCKTAIL Peanuts, chopped

Instructions:

Pour teriyaki sauce over tofu in shallow dish. Refrigerate 10 min. Drain tofu, reserving the teriyaki sauce.

Heat oil in large skillet on medium heat. Add tofu; cook 3 to 4 min. or until golden brown on all sides, stirring occasionally. Remove tofu from skillet.

Add peppers to skillet; cook and stir 2 min. Add onions; cook and stir 1 min. Add rice and pineapple; mix lightly. Cook 2 to 3 min. or until heated through, stirring frequently. Add nuts, tofu and reserved teriyaki sauce; mix lightly. Cook 2 to 3 min. or until heated through, stirring occasionally.

KETO EGG MUFFINS RECIPE

Ingredients:

- 6 eggs

- 1 scallion

- 5 oz. cooked bacon

- 3 oz. shredded cheese

- 1 tablespoon of red or green pesto

- salt and pepper

Instructions:

Preheat the oven to 350 degrees F. and place muffin cups in baking pan. Chop the scallions and bacon and in a bowl whisk eggs with pesto and seasoning. Add cheese. Scoop batter into muffing cups and add bacon. Bake muffins for 15-20 minutes.

TURKEY OR BEEF CHILI

Ingredients:

- 2 pounds of ground beef or turkey

- 8 cups spinach

- 1 cup tomato sauce

- 2 medium green peppers

- 2/3 medium onion

- 1 tablespoon olive oil

- 1 tablespoon cumin

- 1.5 tablespoons chili powder

- 2 teaspoons cayenne pepper

- 1 teaspoon garlic powder

- salt and pepper

Instructions:

Chop the onion and bell pepper. Add olive oil to a pot and cook beef or turkey until browned. While meat is cooking, saute vegetable in a separate pan with olive oil. Season both the meat and veggies with salt and pepper. Add cumin, chili powder, garlic powder, and cayenne pepper to meat. Once the meat is cooked, add spinach and let it cook for 2-3 minutes. Add tomato sauce to the pot and cook for 10 minutes. Add cooked vegetables and stir well.

CAULIFLOWER-CRUST PIZZA

Ingredients:

- 2 cups cauliflower rice

- 2 tablespoons coconut oil

- 1 teaspoon dried oregano

- 1 teaspoon garlic powder

- 1 large egg white

- 1 cup shredded mozzarella cheese

- 3/4 cup grated parmesan cheese

- 1/2 teaspoon salt

- 1/4 cup marinara

- 1/2 cup grated mozzarella cheese (for topping)

- 3 oz. pepperoni slices (optional)

- 1-2 tablespoons basil leaves (garnish)

- 1 tablespoon olive oil (garnish)

Instructions:

Preheat oven to 400 degrees F. Grate parmesan and mozzarella cheese into a bowl. Keep some cheese on the side for topping. Heat a large pan with coconut oil and add cauli-rice. Season with salt and cook for 15 minutes. Remove from heat and place cauli-rice into a bowl. Add 1 cup of mozzarella and 3/4 cup of parmesan cheese to rice. Also add garlic powder, dried oregano, and one egg white. Combine and mix well with hands. Flatten this dough onto parchment paper on a pizza tray and brush on coconut oil. Bake dough in oven for 15-20 minutes before flipping it over to cook the other side for 10 additional minutes. When the dough is cooked, spread marinara sauce on top and add remaining mozzarella and parmesan cheese on top. Top with pepperoni slices if want and cook the pizza for 5-10 minutes until cheese has melted.

COCONUT CHOCOLATE BARS

Ingredients:

- 1 cup shredded, unsweetened coconut

- 1 packet or 1/2 teaspoon Stevia

- 1 teaspoon vanilla extract

- 1/3 cup coconut cream

- 4 tablespoons coconut oil

- 2 tablespoons unsweetened cocoa powder

- 2 oz. cocoa butter

Instructions:

Mix shredded coconut with coconut cream, half of the vanilla extract and half of the Stevia. Blend well and place the mixture on a small cookie sheet lined with parchment paper. Shape the mixture into a rectangle and place in the freezer for two hours. Remove from the freezer and cut into five bars. While waiting for the bars to freeze cook the chocolate topping: melt coconut oil in a pan and add cocoa powder and remaining Stevia and vanilla extract. Mix on low heat for two minutes. Let the mixture cool to room temperature. Dip frozen bars into the chocolate and coat on both side. Place coated bars back on the cookie sheet and place in fridge until they harden and are ready to enjoy.

CRISPY AND CREAMY PANEER KEBABS

Ingredients:

- 100gms Paneer

- 25gms flaxseed powder

- 30ml coconut milk

- 3tsp ghee

- 1tbsp mint chutney

Instructions:

Cut paneer into thick slices.

Apply mint chutney on one side of two paneer slices and close like a sandwich.

Put coconut milk and flaxseed powder in two separate bowls.

Add salt and pepper to the flaxseed powder as per your taste.

Take each paneer sandwich and dip in coconut milk.

Dab coconut milk dipped paneer sandwich in flaxseed powder on all sides.

Brush some ghee on the non stick grill pan and keep it on medium heat.

Place paneer slices on the heated grill and cook on medium heat.

Flip them over to cook from all sides.

Serve when paneer gets crispy with rich golden color from outside.

CRISPY PANEER KABAB

Ingredients:

- 1.5kg chicken broiler

- 150gms yogurt

- 5tsp ginger and garlic paste

- 30gms onion paste

- 15tsp ghee

- 1 cup cilantro or dhaniya leaves

- 30 gms curry leaves

- 1tsp mustard seeds

- 1tsp table salt

- ½ tsp pink salt

- 1tsp turmeric or haldi powder

- 1tsp red chili powder (optional)

- 2 to 3 green chillies (optional)

Instructions:

Wash chicken and pat dry.

Mix hung curd, turmeric powder, and both the salts. Marinate chicken evenly in that mixture.

Grind onions into fine paste and apply it to chicken. Let it set for 4-5 hours.

After 4-5 hours, heat ghee in the wok.

Add mustard seeds and let them splatter, add curry leaves on a medium heat.

Add chicken and continue cooking on medium heat.

After some time, chicken will start leaving water and will also appear a little tender.

Grind fresh cilantro or dhaniya with green chillies to make a fine paste using water.

Add this paste to the chicken and keep cooking for another 10-15 minutes.

Once all the water in chicken dries it means its cooked and ready for serving.

KETO BULLET PROOF COFFEE

Ingredients:

- Instant coffee

- Cooking coconut oil

- Stevia drops

Instructions:

Boil a mug of water and add 1 tsp of instant coffee in it.

Once the coffee starts boiling, add half tsp coconut oil to it (you can add up to 1 tsp coconut oil as per your taste).

Let it simmer for a few mins before straining in a cup.

Add artificial sweetener of your choice and sip slowly.

Note: Coconut oil can be replaced with ghee or butter in the same quantity.

KETO SUPER ENERGY BAR

Ingredients:

- 100ml coconut oil

- 100gms almonds

- 30gms ground flax seeds

- 15gms chia seeds

- 1scoop MuscleBlaze Whey Protein Powder

- pink salt (optional)

Instructions:

Place a thick bottomed pan on medium heat and pour coconut oil in it.

Grind almonds and put them in heated oil, keep stirring.

Add sweetener and keep stirring on low heat. If you feel that the oil is getting super hot, switch off the heat for three to four minutes.

Add grounded flax seeds and keep stirring.

At last add whey protein and stir to make mixture look nice and sticky.

Add Chia seeds to the pan, mix well and remove from heat.

Line baking tin with parchment or butter paper and put the mixture in it.

Keep the tin in the deep freezer for at least two hours.

Once its set it will come out nicely from the tin.

Cut them into small cubes and store in an air tight container in refrigerator.

CABBAGE NOODLE TUNA CASSEROLE

Prep Time: 15 minutes

Cook Time: 30 minutes

Ingredients:

- 2 tbsp olive oil

- 2 tbsp grass-fed butter

- medium head green cabbage (about 1 1/2 lbs), cut into large shreds

- 1 cup onion, chopped

- 3 ribs celery, chopped

- 2 cloves garlic, minced

- sea salt and black pepper, to taste

- 2 tsp dried dill or 2 tbsp fresh dill

- 2 tsp dry mustard powder

- 2 tbsp lemon zest

- juice of 1 lemon

- 1 1/2 cup heavy cream

- 1 1/4 cup Parmesan cheese, grated, divided

- 3 – 5oz cans albacore tuna, drained

- 1/2 cup frozen peas

Instructions:

Heat the olive oil and butter in an extra large ovenproof skillet over medium heat.

Once heated, add the cabbage, onion, celery, garlic, sea salt and black pepper to the pan.

Sauté until the vegetables are crisp tender – about 10 minutes.

Mix in the dill, mustard powder, lemon zest, and lemon juice.

Pour the heavy cream and 1 cup Parmesan cheese into the pan. Mix in and keep stirring until the cheese has melted and combined with the heavy cream.

Reduce heat to medium low and let simmer to allow the sauce to thicken.

Once the sauce has started to thicken, stir in the tuna and the peas.

Sprinkle the remaining Parmesan over the top of the dish and transfer to the oven.

Broil on high for 3-5 minutes or until the Parmesan on top has made a golden brown crust.

KETO CHIPOTLE RED PEPPER CHEESE DIP

Preparation time: 10 minutes

Cooking time: 20 minutes

Total time: 30minutes

Ingredients (makes about 2 cups/ 6 servings):

- 3 medium red peppers, seeds and stalks removed (400 g/ 14 oz)

- 1 tbsp olive oil (15 ml)

- 1/4 cup sun-dried tomatoes (28 g/ 1 oz)

- 1/3 cup full-fat cream cheese (85 g/ 3 oz)

- 1 garlic clove, minced

- 1 tsp paprika

- pinch of dried chipotle or chile flakes

- sea salt, to taste

- Optional: 1 tsp lemon juice, black pepper and chopped parsley

Instructions:

Preheat the oven to 200 °C/ 400 °F. Remove the stalk and seeds from the peppers. Chop into quarters and place on a baking tray. Drizzle with 1 tbsp of olive oil and roast in the oven for 15 minutes until soft. Keto Chipotle Red Pepper Cheese Dip

Immediately place in a sealable bag and allow to steam naturally for 3-5 minutes. This makes the skins easy to remove. Keto Chipotle Red Pepper Cheese Dip

Peel off the skins. Add the peppers, sun dried tomatoes, chipotle or chilli, paprika, cream cheese, garlic and salt to a mixing bowl. Keto Chipotle Red Pepper Cheese Dip

Blitz with a hand blender until smooth. Place in the fridge to thicken. Optionally, stir through 1 tsp of lemon juice before serving. Keto Chipotle Red Pepper Cheese Dip

Top with cracked black pepper and parsley if you prefer. Serve with crudités or keto crackers. Store in an airtight container in the fridge for up to 2 days.

LOW-CARB TURKISH EGGS

Turkish eggs are a popular breakfast recipe and a low-carb option made with kale and red onion.

Eggs should be part of a healthy keto diet - they are nature's perfect food. Eggs are zero-carb, high in micronutrients such as choline and vitamin B12, and they are also a good source of quality protein.

Kale is a great source of vitamin A, C and potassium and is perfect for those who watch their carb intake. Finally, avocado is the ultimate anti keto-flu food. It's one of the best sources of potassium, a good source of magnesium, and monounsaturated fats which are known to protect against heart disease.

The paprika, chili grass-fed butter drizzle makes it a flavour bomb against the soft egg yolks and creamy yogurt. A super easy, one pot classic that's perfect for a late brunch.

Hands-on: 20 minutes

Overall: 20 minutes

Ingredients (makes 4 servings):

Yogurt topping:

- 1/2 cup + 1 tbsp full-fat yogurt (140 g/ 5 oz)

- 1 tsp each lemon zest and lemon juice

- 1 garlic clove, minced

- 1 tbsp chopped cilantro

- sea salt, to taste

- 1 tsp extra virgin olive oil

Eggs:

- 2 tbsp butter or ghee (28 g/ 1 oz)

- 1 medium red onion, sliced (100 g/ 3.5 oz)

- 200 g finely chopped kale (7 oz)

- 1 tbsp butter or ghee (14 g/ 0.5 oz)

- 4 large eggs

Spicy butter sauce:

- 2 tbsp butter or ghee (28 g/ 1 oz)

- 1/2 tsp paprika

- 1 tsp chili or tomato flakes

Topping:

- 1/2 medium avocado, sliced (75 g/ 2.5 oz)

- 1/4 tsp black pepper

- chili flakes and sea salt, to taste

- 2 tbsp pine nuts (17 g/ 0.6 oz)

Instructions:

Mix all the yogurt ingredients together in a small bowl and set aside: yogurt, lemon juice and zest, garlic, cilantro, salt and olive oil.

Heat 1 oz butter in a cast iron pan. Fry the onions on a low-medium heat for 2 minutes until soft.

Add the kale and cook for a further 2 minutes. Stir to combine.

Make 4 wells in the mixture. Add a small knob of butter (total of about 1/2 oz) to each hole to prevent sticking.

Crack open the eggs, one into each well. Allow to cook for 6 – 8 minutes until the egg whites are set and the yolks soft, or to your liking. Remove from the heat.

In a separate saucepan, melt the remaining 1 oz butter and add the paprika, chilli or tomato flakes and a pinch of salt. Simmer for 30 seconds until bubbling. Remove from the heat.

Top the eggs with sliced avocado and yogurt.

Drizzle with spiced butter and sprinkle with pine nuts. Season with extra salt, pepper and chili flakes.

Drizzle with Sriracha sauce and serve immediately!

SHRIMP TACO BOWLS

Prep Time 15 minutes

Cook Time 5 minutes

Total Time 20 minutes

Ingredients:

Marinade:

- 1 lb medium shrimp peeled and deveined

- 2 tbsp lemon juice

- 2 cloves garlic crushed

- 1 tsp cumin

- 1/8 teaspoon chili powder

- 1 tbsp olive oil

- 1/2 tsp salt

To Serve:

- cilantro leaves

- 1 avocado chopped

Mango salsa:

- 1/2 mango chopped

- 1 cup cherry tomatoes

- 1/2 cup red onion chopped

- 2 tsp lime juice, or to taste salt, to taste

Instructions:

Peel and devein the shrimp.

Add the peeled deveined shrimp to the shrimp taco bowl marinade for 15 minutes.

In the same pan add the shrimp and cook for about two minutes per side or until they turn pink.

Serve with chopped avocado, and make a simple mango salsa with the mango, tomatoes, and onion.

BLACKENED SHRIMP

Prep Time: 5 minutes

Cook Time: 5 minutes

Total Time: 10 minutes

Servings: 4

Calories: 175 kcal

Ingredients:

- 1 lb shrimp peeled, deveined

- 3 tbsp homemade Blackened Seasoning

- 2 tbsp olive oil

Instructions:

Toss peeled and deveined shrimp with the blackened seasoning and let sit in the fridge for 10-15 minutes.

Heat the oil in a wide skillet.

Cook the shrimp for about 2 minutes and then turn them over for a couple more minutes until they are cooked all the way through, they will turn pink/white color when they are done.

PARMESAN CARROTS

Prep Time: 10 minutes

Cook Time: 20 minutes

Total Time: 30 minutes

Ingredients:

- 1 lb carrots peeled and cut into sticks

- 2 tbsp olive oil

- 2 cloves garlic crushed

- 1/4 tsp black pepper ground

- 1/2 tsp salt

- 3 tbsp Parmesan cheese grated

Instructions:

Preheat the oven to 400F.

Line a sheet pan with parchment paper.

Toss carrots in olive oil, garlic, salt and pepper.

Bake for 15 minutes then sprinkle on the Parmesan cheese.

Bake for a further 5-10 minutes until carrots are soft and the cheese is melted.

Remove from the oven and serve hot.

CHICKEN AVOCADO SALAD

This Chicken Avocado Salad with Honey-Lime Dressing is such a fun summer salad! It's jam-packed with healthy ingredients including arugula, spinach, and mango.

Prep Time: 10 minutes

Cook Time: 10 minutes

Total Time: 20 minutes

Ingredients:

- 2 cups Romaine lettuce

- 1 cup arugula

- 1 cup baby spinach

- 1 avocado

- 1/2 English cucumber

- 1 cup cherry tomatoes

- 1 cup mango

- 1/2 cup red onion chopped

Chicken marinade:

- 4 chicken thighs skinless and boneless

- 1 lime zest from one lime

- 3 tbsp fresh lime juice approx two limes

- 3 tbsp olive oil

- 4 cloves garlic crushed

- 2 tsp oregano

- 1/2 tsp salt

- 1/2 tsp pepper

Honey-lime dressing:

- 3 tablespoons olive oil

- 2 tbsp fresh lime juice approx 1 lime

- 2 tsp honey

- 1/2 tsp salt

- 1/8th tsp cayenne pepper

Instructions:

Mix together the grilled chicken marinade and pour over the chicken. Marinate for 1 hour.

Cook the chicken on a grill or in a cast iron grill pan with a little oil on a medium heat until it's cooked all the way through.

To make the honey-lime dressing mix all the ingredients together to combine. taste and adjust the seasonings and honey if you need to.

Assemble your chicken avocado salad by adding the romaine lettuce, arugula, baby spinach, grilled chicken, avocado, cucumber, cherry tomatoes, mango, and red onion into a large bowl. Add as much salad dressing as you like, then toss salad.

ULTIMATE KETO BUNS

Hands-on: 10-15 minutes

Overall: 55-60 minutes

Ingredients (makes 10 buns):

Dry ingredients:

- 1 1/2 cup almond flour (almond meal) (150 g/ 5.3 oz)

- 2/3 cup psyllium husks - will be powdered, or 1/3 cup psyllium husk powder (40 g/ 1.4 oz)

- 1/2 cup coconut flour (60 g/ 2.1 oz)

- 1/2 packed cup flax meal (75 g/ 2.6 oz)

- 2 tsp garlic powder

- 2 tsp onion powder

- 2 tsp cream of tartar or apple cider vinegar

- 1 tsp baking soda

- 1 tsp pink Himalayan or sea salt

- 5 tbsp sesame seeds (or sunflower, flax, poppy seeds) or 1-2 tbsp caraway seeds

- Optional: 1-2 tbsp Erythritol or Swerve

Wet ingredients:

- 6 large egg whites

- 2 large eggs

- 2 cups water, boiling or lukewarm depending on the method - see intro (480 ml/ 16 fl oz)

Tips & substitutions:

If making a loaf instead of buns, bake for 75 minutes! Do not use a silicon loaf pan - use a metallic one instead.

Flax-free, multi-purpose bread, includes a nut-free option.

Nut-free keto buns - include flaxmeal

If you don't want to use coconut flour: use twice the amount of almond flour or flaxmeal instead of coconut flour (1 cup of almond flour/flaxmeal instead of 1/2 cup coconut flour). Or you can use the same amount but reduce the water by 1/2 cup.

If using apple cider vinegar instead of cream of tartar, make sure to mix it with the wet ingredients.

For best results, use a kitchen scale when measuring all the dry ingredients. Using just cups may not be enough to achieve best results, especially in baked goods. Weights per cups and tablespoons may vary depending on the product/ brand or if you make you own ingredients (like flaxmeal from flaxseeds). Psyllium absorbs lots of water.

When baking with psyllium, you must remember to drink enough water throughout the day to prevent constipation.

Instructions:

Preheat the oven to 175 °C/ 350 °F. Use a kitchen scale to measure all the ingredients and add them to a mixing bowl (apart from the sesame seeds which are used for topping): almond flour, coconut flour, flax meal, psyllium husk powder, garlic powder, onion powder, cream of tartar, baking soda, salt (and optionally, Erythritol).

Do not use whole psyllium husks - if you cannot find psyllium husk powder, use a blender or coffee grinder and process until fine. If you get already prepared psyllium husk powder, remember to weigh it before adding to the recipe. I used whole psyllium husks which I powdered myself. Do not use just measuring cups - different products have different weights per cup!

Mix all the dry ingredients.

Cream of tartar and baking soda act as leavening agents. This is how it works: To get 2 teaspoons of gluten-free baking powder, you need 1/2 a teaspoon of baking soda and 1 teaspoon of cream of tartar (double in this recipe of 10 buns). If you don't have cream of tartar, instead you can use apple cider vinegar and add it to the wet ingredients.

Erythritol could be omitted in this recipe - the effect on carbs is minimum. It works in two ways: it acts as leavening agent and creates the slightly sweet taste burger buns have. Also, if you don't have both onion and garlic powder, you can use just one of them or use freshly mashed garlic cloves (2 cloves per recipe of 5 buns).

Add the egg whites and eggs. and process well using a mixer until the dough is thick.

The reason you shouldn't use only whole eggs is that the buns wouldn't rise with so many egg yolks in. Don't waste them - use them for making Home-made Mayo, Easy Hollandaise Sauce or Lemon Curd.

Add boiling water and process until well combined.

Using a spoon, make the buns and place them on a non-stick baking tray or a parchment paper. They will grow in size, so make sure to leave some space between them. You can even use small tart trays.

Top each of the buns with sesame seeds (or any other seeds) and press them into the dough, so they don't fall out. Place in the oven and cook for 45-50 minutes.

Remove from the oven, let the tray cool down and place the buns on a rack to cool down to room temperature. Store them at room temperature if you plan to use them in the next couple of days or store in the freezer for future use.

Top with butter or cream cheese, burger meat or any topping you like.

Tip: To save time, mix all the dry ingredients ahead and store in a zip-lock bag and add a label with the number of servings. When ready to be baked, just add the wet ingredients!

Suggestions:

If for any reason you can't get this recipe to work, here are some tips that might help. Most of the above tips apply to any recipes using psyllium husk powder:

Make sure you weigh all the ingredients using scales. Even small differences can affect the final result of this recipe.

If the buns appear to have large hollow bubbles inside, it may be due to the psyllium. Make sure you use powder, not whole husks. Otherwise, use a coffee grinder or blender and pulse until fine and powdery.

For a slightly (but not significantly) better result, incorporate the eggs separately. First, whisk the egg whites until they create soft peaks and add cream of tartar used in this recipe. In another bowl, mix the egg yolks and gently fold them into the egg whites. In a separate bowl, mix the dry ingredients and pour in the hot water. Process well using an electric mixer (hand whisk is not as good in this recipe). Add the foamy egg white mixture into the batter and process well. Try not to deflate the batter completely. Form the buns and place in the oven.

If the buns don't rise properly, use only egg whites and omit the egg yolks.

If the final result is too moist, do not reduce the water used in this recipe or the psyllium will clump. Instead, dry the buns in the oven on low, up to 100 °C/ 210 °F for 30-60 minutes. If needed, cut them in half and place in a toaster.

Do not leave the batter outside the oven for too long. Place in the oven as soon as you form the buns.

If the buns change color to slight purple, it's due to the psyllium husk powder. Whenever I use whole husks and grind them at home, they are always perfect, light brown. However, when I use ready-made psyllium husk powder, they look purple, especially the next day. Although they may not look appetising, they are perfectly fine.

KETO RASPBERRY LEMON LOAF

Hands-on: 10 minutes

Overall: 1 hour 10 minutes

Ingredients (10 servings):

Loaf:

- 3 large eggs

- 1 large egg white

- juice and zest from 1 lemon

- 1/4 cup melted butter, ghee or virgin coconut oil (60 ml/ 2 fl oz)

- 1 1/2 cups almond flour (150 g/ 5.3 oz)

- 3/4 cup powdered Swerve (108 g/ 3.8 oz)

- 1/4 tsp sea salt

- 1 tsp baking powder

- 1 cup fresh raspberries (120 g/ 4.2 oz)

Glaze & topping:

- 1/2 cup powdered Swerve (80 g/ 2.8 oz)

- juice and zest from 1 lemon

- 1/2 cup fresh raspberries (62 g/ 2.2 oz)

Note: The glaze is very sweet and may be too sweet for those who are used to low-carb eating. Alternatively, you can use the glaze in our Low-Carb Lemon Cake which is made with melted coconut butter, coconut oil, lemon juice and lemon zest (sweetener can be skipped or used to taste).

Instructions:

Preheat oven to 175 °C/ 350 °F and line a loaf pan with parchment paper.

In a large bowl whisk together the dry cake ingredients. In another bowl, beat the eggs using a hand mixer.

Add the melted butter (or ghee), lemon juice, and lemon zest.

Gently fold in the raspberries and mix using a spatula.

Pour into the loaf pan lined with parchment paper and spread evenly using a spatula.

Bake for 1 hour or until a toothpick inserted into the center comes out clean. Once cooked, remove from the oven, set aside and let cool before adding the glaze.

To make the glaze simply mix together the ingredients in a small bowl until smooth.

Pour over the cooled loaf.

Sprinkle with the reserved raspberries.

Slice and serve. Store covered in the refrigerator for up to 5 days.

CONCLUSION

Start burning fat today without more exercise! Take control of your metabolism naturally by adopting a ketogenic diet plan. Your body was designed for this style of nutrition. Your metabolic state can be optimized by consuming the (delicious) foods that our genetic forefathers thrived on, and this does not include carbohydrate-rich, processed foods loaded with sugars and bad fats. It involves a luxurious and fulfilling diet based on bountiful foods from paleolithic times, including lean meats, vegetables, nuts and seeds, and healthy fats that your body will thank you for.

Virtually all weight loss diets to varying degrees focus on either calorie reduction or the manipulation of the intake of one of the three essential macronutrients (proteins, fats, or carbohydrates) to achieve their weight loss effects.

Ketogenic diets are a group of "high-fat, moderate protein" or "high-protein moderate fat" but very low-carbohydrate diets. The term ketogenic basically refers to the increased production of ketone bodies occasioned by the elevated rate of lipolysis (fat break down). Ketones are acidic by-products formed during the intermediate break down of "fat" into "fatty acids" by the liver.

Despite the ability of ketogenic diets to reduce insulin production, their main objective is ultimately aimed at inducing the state of ketosis. Ketosis can be regarded as a condition or state in which the rate of formation of ketones produced by the break-down of "fat" into "fatty acids" by the liver is greater than the ability of tissues to oxidize them. Ketosis is actually a secondary state of the process of lipolysis (fat break down) and is a general side effect of low-carbohydrate diets. Ketogenic diets are therefore favorably disposed to the encouragement and promotion of ketosis.

Prolonged periods of starvation can easily induce ketosis but they can also be deliberately induced by making use of a low-calorie or low-carbohydrate diet through the ingestion of large amounts of either fats or proteins and drastically reduced carbohydrates. Therefore, high-fat and high-protein diets are the weight loss diets used to deliberately induce ketosis.

Essentially, ketosis is a very efficient form of energy production which does not involve the production of insulin as the body rather burns its fat deposits for energy. Consequently, the idea of reducing carbohydrate consumption does not only reduce insulin production but also practically forces the body to burn its fat deposit for energy, thereby making use of ketogenic diets is a very powerful way to achieve rapid weight loss.

Ketogenic diets are designed in such a way that they initially force the body to exhaust its glucose supply and then finally switch to burning its fat deposits for energy. Subsequent food intakes after inducing the state of ketosis are meant to keep the ketosis process running by appropriately adjusting further carbohydrate consumption to provide just the basic amount of calories needed by the body.

9 781801 446266